BODYBUILDING 101

The Basics of Sculpting Your Perfect Physique

Philipp Frühwirth

CONTENTS

WHAT IS BODYBUILDING AND WHY IS IT IMPORTANT?

Bodybuilding is a sport that involves the intentional growth and shaping of muscles through resistance training and proper nutrition. While bodybuilding is often associated with competitive bodybuilding events, many people engage in the sport simply for its physical and mental health benefits.

At its core, bodybuilding is all about hard work, patience, and discipline. By working the muscles to their limits through exercise and focusing on nutrition, bodybuilders can achieve impressive results, such as increased muscle mass, improved strength and endurance, and a leaner physique.

But bodybuilding offers much more than just physical benefits. The practice of bodybuilding can also have positive effects on mental health, such as reducing stress and anxiety, increasing confidence, and promoting a healthy body image.

For many people, bodybuilding serves as an important means of self-expression and personal growth. Through bodybuilding, individuals can challenge themselves to push beyond their limits, set and achieve ambitious goals, and grow as individuals.

In addition to physical and mental benefits, bodybuilding can also have a positive impact on overall health. Regular exercise has been linked to reduced risk of chronic disease, improved cardiovascular health, and increased longevity.

Bodybuilding also offers a number of practical benefits. By increasing strength and endurance, bodybuilders can perform everyday tasks with greater ease and efficiency. Additionally, bodybuilding can help to prevent injury by strengthening muscles and bones, improving balance and coordination, and enhancing overall physical fitness.

In short, bodybuilding is an impactful sport that offers numerous benefits to those who practice it. Whether you are a seasoned athlete or just starting out, incorporating bodybuilding into your fitness routine can help you achieve your goals, both physically and mentally. With dedication, discipline, and hard work, you can improve your overall health and achieve a stronger, leaner, and more confident body.

THE BENEFITS OF BODYBUILDING FOR A HEALTHY LIFESTYLE

Bodybuilding is more than just an activity to improve your physique. It also provides numerous benefits for a healthy lifestyle. Here are some of the major benefits of bodybuilding:

1. Increased Muscle Mass: A major benefit of bodybuilding is that it helps increase muscle mass. This is important as muscle helps you burn more calories and fat while at rest, thus improving your overall metabolism. Moreover, increased muscle mass contributes to better posture, strength, and endurance.
2. Reduced Risk of Chronic Diseases: Studies have found that bodybuilding can reduce the risk of chronic diseases such as heart disease, stroke, and some forms of cancer. This is because physical activity helps keep your cardiovascular system healthy and reduces inflammation in the body.
3. Improved Mental Health: Bodybuilding has also been linked to improved mental health. Working out releases endorphins, the "feel-good" hormones, which can help reduce symptoms of depression and anxiety. In addition, bodybuilding can improve confidence, self-esteem, and overall mood.
4. Better Insulin Sensitivity: Insulin sensitivity refers to how well your body uses insulin to convert glucose (sugar) to energy. Bodybuilding has been shown to improve insulin sensitivity, which is beneficial for individuals with diabetes or pre-diabetes.
5. Increased Bone Density: Bodybuilding can help increase bone density, which is particularly important as we age. This reduces the risk of osteoporosis and other bone-related injuries.
6. Enhanced Sleep: Regular exercise including bodybuilding can

improve sleep quality and regulate sleep-wake cycles. This has positive effects on overall health, including immune system function and mood.

In addition to these benefits, bodybuilding can also help individuals build a strong support system and improve their social connections. It can be a great way to meet like-minded individuals who share a passion for fitness and a healthy lifestyle.

Overall, bodybuilding can be a powerful tool for improving health and achieving a strong, well-toned physique. Incorporating bodybuilding into your exercise routine can provide a wide range of benefits that extend beyond the physical, ultimately contributing to a healthier and happier life.

HOW TO DETERMINE YOUR BODYBUILDING GOALS

Having clear goals is essential to success in any endeavor, and bodybuilding is no exception. Without a well-defined objective, it's easy to lose direction and motivation. But how do you determine your bodybuilding goals? The following tips can help:

1. Assess your current physique: Before you can set meaningful goals, you need to know where you're starting from. Take measurements of your body fat percentage, muscle mass, and other relevant metrics. This will give you a baseline to work from and allow you to track your progress.

2. Define your priorities: What is most important to you? Is it building muscle mass, losing body fat, or improving overall fitness? Your goals should align with your personal values and aspirations.

3. Be specific: Vague goals like "getting in shape" are hard to measure and unlikely to motivate you. Set concrete, specific targets, such as increasing your bench press by 20 pounds or reducing your body fat percentage by 5%.

4. Make your goals realistic: While it's important to challenge yourself, setting unattainable goals can be discouraging. Consider your current fitness level, lifestyle constraints, and other factors when setting your objectives.

5. Set a timeline: Goals without deadlines are just wishes. Determine when you want to achieve your objectives and create a timeline with milestones along the way. This will help you stay on track and celebrate your accomplishments.

6. Write it down: There's a powerful psychological effect to writing down your goals. Put your objectives on paper, including your reasons for pursuing them, and review them regularly to stay focused and motivated.

7. Get professional guidance: If you're new to bodybuilding or uncertain about how to set goals, consider working with a personal trainer or other fitness professional. They can help you assess your current condition, clarify your objectives, and develop a personalized plan to achieve them.

Setting clear and achievable goals is the foundation of success in bodybuilding. Take the time to assess your current situation, define your priorities, and create a specific, measurable plan for achieving your objectives. With persistence and dedication, you can transform your body and achieve your dreams.

THE SCIENCE OF MUSCLE BUILDING AND EXERCISE PHYSIOLOGY

Muscle building, also known as hypertrophy, is the process of increasing muscle size through resistance training and proper nutrition. Understanding the science of muscle building and exercise physiology can help improve your workout routine and optimize your results.

Muscles are made up of muscle fibers, which are organized into bundles. These fibers consist of two types of proteins: myosin and actin. When a muscle is activated, these two proteins interact to create force and movement.

Resistance training, such as weight lifting or bodyweight exercises, creates small microscopic tears in muscle fibers. The body then repairs these tears, resulting in an increase in muscle size and strength. This process is known as muscle hypertrophy.

To achieve hypertrophy, it's important to perform exercises that target specific muscle groups. This often involves focusing on compound exercises that work multiple muscle groups simultaneously, such as squats, deadlifts, and bench press. Isolation exercises, which target a specific muscle group, can also be used to supplement compound exercises.

To continue to make progress, it's important to challenge your muscles through progressive overload. This involves gradually increasing weight, reps, or sets over time to continually stimulate muscle growth.

Nutrition also plays a crucial role in muscle building. Adequate protein intake is essential for muscle recovery and growth. The recommended daily intake for protein is generally around 1 gram per pound of body weight.

Carbohydrates and fats are also important for providing energy during workouts and supporting overall health. Complex carbohydrates, such as whole grains and vegetables, are typically the best choice for fueling workouts, while healthy fats, such as those found in nuts and avocados, can provide essential nutrients and promote satiety.

Rest and recovery are equally important aspects of muscle building. Adequate rest helps the body repair and rebuild muscle tissue, and prevents overtraining and burnout. It's also important to vary your workouts and allow time for active recovery, such as stretching or light cardio.

In conclusion, muscle building is a complex process that involves both exercise and nutrition. Understanding the science behind muscle building can help you optimize your workouts and achieve your goals. By incorporating progressive overload, proper nutrition, and adequate rest and recovery, you can enhance your muscle building efforts and improve your overall health and fitness.

CREATING A BALANCED AND EFFECTIVE BODYBUILDING WORKOUT PLAN

If you want to see results from bodybuilding, it's important to have a well-rounded workout plan that targets all major muscle groups in your body. Here are some tips for creating a balanced and effective bodybuilding workout plan:

1. Determine your training split
The first step in creating a workout plan is deciding how many days per week you will be training, and how you will split your workouts. The most common training splits include:

- Full body: Training all major muscle groups in one workout, usually 2-3 times per week
- Upper/Lower: Training upper body and lower body on different days, usually 4 times per week
- Push/Pull/Legs: Training push muscles (chest, shoulders, triceps), pull muscles (back, biceps), and legs on different days, usually 5-6 times per week

Choose a training split that fits your schedule and goals.

2. Choose your exercises
Next, choose exercises that target each major muscle group. Examples include:

- Chest: Bench press, incline press, flyes
- Back: Pull-ups, rows, lat pulldowns
- Shoulders: Overhead press, lateral raises, reverse flyes
- Biceps: Curls, hammer curls, chin-ups
- Triceps: Dips, skullcrushers, close-grip bench press

- Legs: Squats, deadlifts, lunges, leg curls, calf raises

Include a variety of exercises that target different aspects of each muscle group (e.g. incline bench press targets the upper chest, while flyes target the lower chest).

3. Determine your sets and reps
Each exercise should be performed for 3-4 sets of 8-15 reps. Heavy weight and lower reps (3-5) can be used for strength training, while lighter weight and higher reps (15-20) are often used for endurance training.

4. Plan your rest periods
Rest periods between sets should be 1-2 minutes for hypertrophy (muscle growth) and 3-5 minutes for strength training.

5. Incorporate progressive overload
Progressive overload is the key to muscle growth. It involves gradually increasing the weight or reps you use for each exercise over time. This can be done by increasing weight, reps, or reducing rest periods as you get stronger.

6. Don't forget about cardio
While building muscle is important for bodybuilding, cardio is also important for overall health and fitness. Include 20-30 minutes of moderate intensity cardio (e.g. jogging, cycling) after your weight lifting workouts.

By following these tips, you can create a balanced and effective bodybuilding workout plan that targets all major muscle groups and helps you reach your fitness goals.

NUTRITION FOR BODYBUILDING: THE ESSENTIAL MACROS AND MICROS

Nutrition plays a crucial role in bodybuilding. It's essential to consume the right nutrients in the right amounts to build muscle, maintain energy levels, and support overall health. Macros and micros are the two types of nutrients that make up our daily diet. In this chapter, we'll take a look at the essential macros and micros that every bodybuilder needs.

Macros, short for macronutrients, are the primary sources of energy for the body. They consist of carbohydrates, proteins, and fats. To build muscle, your body needs an appropriate balance of all three. Proteins are essential for muscle growth and repair, while carbs provide fuel for energy and fats provide long-lasting energy and maintain hormonal balance.

Carbohydrates: Carbohydrates are the body's primary source of energy. They're essential for fueling high-intensity training sessions and replenishing glycogen stores in the muscles. The recommended intake is 2-3 grams per pound of body weight, but it's best to consult with a nutritionist and determine your specific needs based on your training goals.

Proteins: Proteins are the building blocks of muscles. They help repair and rebuild muscle tissue after a workout. The recommended intake is around 1 gram per pound of body weight, but again, it's best to consult with a professional and determine your specific needs.

Fats: Fats are essential for the healthy functioning of the body. They help regulate hormones and maintain the structure and function of cell membranes. A recommended intake of healthy fats is around 0.5 grams per pound of body weight.

Micronutrients or micronutrients include vitamins and minerals that the body needs in small quantities but plays a significant role in maintaining overall health, including supporting the immune system, building strong bones, and regulating crucial functions in the body.

Some of the key micronutrients preferred by bodybuilders include:
- Zinc: Zinc helps to build muscle, maintain hormone levels, and support an immune system.
- Magnesium: Magnesium reduces muscle fatigue, helps with energy production, and prevents muscle cramps.
- Iron: Iron is necessary for the delivery of oxygen to the muscles, which is critical during intense training sessions.
- B-vitamins: B-vitamins are essential for energy production, muscle repair, and recovery.

In conclusion, macros and micros are both critical to a bodybuilder's diet. A balance of carbs, protein, and fat is necessary for energy and muscle gain, while vitamins and minerals play a significant role in maintaining overall health, which directly affects performance. Consulting with a professional nutritionist is advisable to ensure an optimal diet conducive to achieving bodybuilding goals.

HOW TO BUILD MUSCLE MASS: UNDERSTANDING PROGRESSIVE OVERLOAD

Building muscle mass is one of the primary goals of bodybuilding, and understanding the principle of progressive overload is essential to achieving this goal. Progressive overload refers to the gradual increase of resistance or weight in your workouts over time to continue challenging your muscles and promoting growth.

Here are ways to apply the principle of progressive overload to build muscle mass effectively:

1. Increase Resistance - Gradually increase the amount of resistance or weight you lift during your workouts. This can be done by adding more weights to your machines or free weights or using resistance bands.

2. Increase Volume - Increasing volume refers to performing more sets or reps of an exercise. For example, if you usually perform three sets of ten reps of a particular exercise, you can increase the volume by performing four sets of twelve reps.

3. Decrease Rest - Shortening your rest intervals between sets can add intensity to your workouts, promoting muscle growth. For example, reducing your rest time from two minutes to one minute between sets allows less time for recovery.

4. Increase Frequency - Increasing the frequency of your workouts allows more frequent stimulation of your muscles. It can be beneficial to divide your workouts into different body parts to avoid overtraining.

It is important to incorporate progressive overload gradually and consistently. Aim to increase the resistance, volume or frequency of your workouts every two to four weeks. This gradual increase helps avoid injury or overtraining while providing time for your muscles to adapt and grow.

However, it is essential to ensure sufficient rest and recovery times between workouts. Overtraining can result in severe muscle injury or a lack of gains. Adequate sleep, nutrition, and rest are crucial factors in promoting muscle growth.

In conclusion, progressive overload is essential for building muscle mass in bodybuilding. It is a matter of gradually increasing the resistance, volume, and frequency of your workouts over time. By incorporating this principle, each of your workouts will challenge your muscles and stimulate growth, leading to noticeable gains over time.

THE IMPORTANCE OF REST AND RECOVERY IN BODYBUILDING

One common mistake that many bodybuilders make is not giving their body enough time to rest and recover between workouts. This can lead to overtraining, injuries, and slower muscle growth. Rest and recovery are just as important as the actual workout itself.

Rest and recovery can be achieved in a variety of ways. One popular method is to take rest days, where you avoid any strenuous exercise and instead focus on recovering. Your body needs time to heal and repair the damage that occurs during intense exercise. During rest days, you can take the time to stretch, do some low-intensity cardio, or participate in other activities that don't put too much stress on your muscles.

Another important factor in rest and recovery is getting enough sleep. Aim for seven to nine hours of quality sleep each night to help your body heal and repair itself. When you sleep, your body produces growth hormone, which helps to repair and regenerate muscle tissue. Getting enough sleep can also help to lower stress levels, which can negatively affect muscle growth.

Another way to promote recovery is through nutrition. Eating a balanced diet that is rich in protein, complex carbohydrates, and healthy fats can help to fuel your muscles and promote their growth and repair. Make sure to eat enough calories to support your workouts and give your body the energy it needs to build muscle.

Lastly, consider incorporating active recovery into your workout routine. This means doing light exercise or stretching on days when you're not working out. This can help to improve blood flow, reduce soreness, and improve flexibility, which can all help to speed up the recovery process.

In conclusion, rest and recovery are essential components of a successful bodybuilding program. Without sufficient rest and recovery, you may not achieve the muscle growth and strength gains you're striving for, and you may even risk injury. Be sure to prioritize rest and recovery as much as you prioritize your workouts, and you'll be on your way to achieving your goals.

THE ROLE OF SUPPLEMENTS IN BODYBUILDING: WHAT WORKS, WHAT DOESN'T?

As you dive deeper into the world of bodybuilding, you'll come across many supplements claiming to help you build muscle and achieve your desired physique. However, not all supplements are created equal, and some may even be harmful if taken improperly. In this chapter, we will take a closer look at the role of supplements in bodybuilding and discuss what works and what doesn't.

Protein Supplements: The Best Bang for Your Buck

Protein is the most essential nutrient for muscle growth, and it's challenging to consume sufficient amounts through food alone. Therefore, protein supplements can be an excellent way to ensure that you're meeting your required protein intake. Whey protein is one of the most popular protein supplements and is an excellent source of protein because it contains all the essential amino acids required for muscle growth.

Creatine: The Most Effective Supplement for Building Muscle

Creatine is one of the most effective supplements for building muscle, and it's backed by plenty of scientific research. It works by increasing phosphocreatine stores in your muscles, which in turn, helps to produce more energy during high-intensity workouts. This results in enhanced muscle growth and increased strength over time. While creatine can provide great benefits, it's important to drink plenty of water to avoid dehydration.

Pre-Workout: Are They Worth It?

Pre-workout supplements usually contain a blend of caffeine, creatine, and other ingredients designed to boost energy and improve performance levels. While these supplements can give you a quick burst of energy, they may also contain high levels of caffeine that can cause nervousness, jitters, and unpleasant side effects. It's crucial to do your research before trying any new supplement, and you always should follow the manufacturer's suggested serving size.

What to Avoid: Questionable and Risky Supplements

While some supplements are safe and effective, others can be downright dangerous. These supplements promise quick weight loss, increased energy or performance, but they usually have little evidence to support their claims. Some of the most risky and ineffective supplements you should avoid in bodybuilding are weight loss pills, testosterone boosters, prohormones, and steroid alternatives.

Conclusion

In conclusion, supplements can be a valuable asset to your bodybuilding routine, but they are not a substitute for a proper diet and workout plan. If you choose to supplement, it's crucial to only purchase from reputable sources, stick to the recommended dosages, and be aware of any side effects or adverse reactions associated with the supplement. Always remember that supplements should only be used to enhance your bodybuilding journey and not replace good old-fashioned hard work and dedication.

INJURY PREVENTION AND CORRECTIVE EXERCISES IN BODYBUILDING

Bodybuilding is an intense sport that requires discipline, dedication, and a relentless focus on progress. However, this focus on continual improvement can often lead to overtraining or poor technique, leading to injury. To avoid these pitfalls, bodybuilders must implement a comprehensive injury prevention program that includes corrective exercises.

Corrective exercises are targeted movements that help identify and address muscular imbalances, which can occur for a variety of reasons, including poor technique, lack of mobility, or compensation for injury. These imbalances can lead to overuse injuries or affect your exercise performance, limiting your progress.

To prevent these issues, bodybuilders should implement exercises that target common areas of weakness, including the hips, shoulders, knees, and core. Here are some corrective exercises that can help:

1. Glute Bridge - This exercise strengthens the glutes, which are often weak due to long periods of sitting. Lie on your back with your knees bent and feet flat on the ground. Drive through your heels and lift your hips off the ground, squeezing your glutes at the top.

2. Face Pulls - This exercise strengthens the upper back and helps correct posture. Attach a resistance band to a stable object at chest height. Hold the band with both hands and pull towards your face, keeping your elbows high and back straight.

3. Planks - This is an essential exercise for strengthening the core muscles. Start in a push-up position but with your forearms on the ground. Keep your body straight and hold for 30-60 seconds.

4. Wall Angels - This exercise helps correct posture and open up the chest. Stand against a wall with your arms bent at a 90-degree angle, palms facing forward. Slowly slide your arms up the wall as high as you can, then return to the starting position.

5. Calf Raises - This exercise strengthens the calves, which can be a weak area for some people. Stand on the edge of a step with your heels hanging off. Rise up onto your toes, then lower back down.

Along with these exercises, bodybuilders should prioritize rest and recovery to prevent injury. Rest days are crucial for allowing the body to recover from intense workouts and repair damaged muscles. Adequate sleep, hydration, and proper nutrition are also essential components of recovery.

In conclusion, bodybuilders must prioritize injury prevention as much as they do strength training. Implementing a corrective exercise routine and prioritizing rest and recovery can help ensure long-term progress and prevent injuries from derailing your journey.

BODYBUILDING AND CARDIO: FINDING THE RIGHT BALANCE

Cardiovascular exercise is an important part of a healthy lifestyle, but for those who are focused on bodybuilding, it can be challenging to find the right balance between cardio and weightlifting. While both forms of exercise have numerous benefits, they can also impact each other in negative ways if not properly coordinated.

Cardio exercise, in general, helps improve heart health, lung capacity, and weight management. Weightlifting, on the other hand, helps to build muscle, strength, and bone density. Bodybuilders want to maintain a low level of body fat to showcase their muscle definition, so cardio can be a useful tool to burn calories and reduce body fat.

However, excessive cardio can also be detrimental to muscle gain as it can interfere with recovery time and hinder the body's ability to build muscle. Excessive cardio can even lead to muscle loss in some cases.

So, how do you find the right balance between cardio and weightlifting? There is no one right answer, and the balance depends on your individual goals, fitness level, and other factors. However, here are some general tips to consider:

1. Determine Your Goals: Before deciding on how much cardio to do, you first need to determine your goals. If you're primarily focused on building muscle and strength, then you may want to minimize cardio to maintain an optimal hormonal environment for muscle growth. If your goals include improving your cardiovascular endurance or losing weight, then you may need to

allocate more time to cardio.

2. Design a Workout Plan: Once you know your goals, you can design a workout plan that incorporates both weightlifting and cardio. Consider the specific types of cardio you enjoy and choose ones that will not interfere with your weightlifting schedule. High-intensity interval training (HIIT) and steady-state cardio are both effective options for bodybuilders.

3. Plan Your Cardio Sessions: Consider adding cardio sessions on days when you are not lifting weights or schedule them after your weightlifting sessions. Avoid doing cardio before weightlifting, as it can lead to fatigue and weaker lifting performance.

4. Monitor Progress: Keep track of how you feel during and after workouts and monitor your progress regularly. If you notice signs of fatigue, overtraining, or lack of results, adjust your plan accordingly.

Finding the right balance between cardio and weightlifting is crucial to achieving your bodybuilding goals. Experiment with different approaches and listen to your body to find the right balance that works for you.

ADVANCED BODYBUILDING TECHNIQUES: DROP SETS, SUPER SETS AND MORE

Once you have mastered the basics of bodybuilding, it's time to take your training to the next level. Advanced bodybuilding techniques can help you to break through plateaus, build muscle more efficiently, and take your physique to the next level. In this chapter, we'll explore some of the most effective advanced bodybuilding techniques, including drop sets, super sets, and more.

Drop Sets

Drop sets are a powerful technique for increasing muscle fatigue and promoting muscle growth. With a drop set, you perform an exercise until you reach muscle failure, then immediately reduce the weight and continue the exercise. This allows you to continue working the muscle while fatigued, pushing it to adapt and grow.

To perform a drop set, start by selecting a weight that is challenging for you to lift for 8-10 reps. Perform the exercise until you reach failure. Reduce the weight by about 20-30% and immediately continue the exercise until failure again. Repeat this process for 2-3 drop sets.

Super Sets

With a super set, you perform two exercises back to back with no rest in between. This technique is great for promoting muscle growth and burning fat, as it increases the intensity of your workout and reduces the time you spend resting.

To perform a super set, select two exercises that work different muscle groups. For example, you could start with a set of bench presses, followed immediately by a set of bent-over rows. Perform each exercise for the desired number of reps, then rest for 60-90 seconds before starting the next set.

Giant Sets

Giant sets are similar to super sets, but instead of two exercises, you perform three or more back to back. This technique is great for targeting a specific muscle group and hitting it from all angles.

To perform a giant set, select three or more exercises that work the same muscle group. For example, you could perform a set of squats, followed by leg press, and finish with lunges. Perform each exercise for the desired number of reps, then rest for 60-90 seconds before starting the next set.

Isometrics

Isometrics are another advanced bodybuilding technique that can help you to increase muscle strength and size. With an isometric, you hold a weight or resistance in a fixed position, without moving.

To perform an isometric, select an exercise and hold the position for 20-30 seconds. For example, you could hold a dumbbell curl halfway through the range of motion, or hold a squat at the bottom of the movement.

Summary

Advanced bodybuilding techniques like drop sets, super sets, giant sets, and isometrics can help you to build muscle more efficiently, break through plateaus, and take your training to the next level. Incorporate these techniques into your workout routine to challenge yourself, increase intensity, and achieve your bodybuilding goals.

HOW TO MEASURE AND TRACK YOUR PROGRESS IN BODYBUILDING

When it comes to bodybuilding, tracking your progress is essential to keep motivation high and reach your goals. Improvement is not only visible in the mirror but also in strength, muscle mass, and body fat levels. In this chapter, we will discuss some of the best ways to measure and track progress in bodybuilding.

1. Bodyweight

One of the simplest and most basic ways to track progress is by measuring your body weight. However, it is essential to understand that bodyweight alone doesn't provide a complete picture of your progress. Bodyweight can fluctuate due to various factors like water retention, food intake, and time of day. For a more accurate measurement, record your weight at the same time of the day, preferably first thing in the morning.

2. Body Measurements

Taking body measurements is an excellent way to track progress, especially if your goal is to lose fat or gain muscle mass. The most common body measurements include waist, hips, thighs, chest, arms, and calves. Taking measurements regularly can help to track the progress of the body parts gaining or losing the most.

3. Progress Photos

Taking progress photos is a great way to visually see your body transformation. Take pictures often (once a week or every two weeks) in the same lighting and position, and compare them side by side. Progress photos can give you a better idea of your body composition changes and help identify weak areas that need more attention.

4. Strength Progression

Strength progression is another fundamental way to track progress in bodybuilding. Keep a record of the weights you use for each exercise and track how they change over time. A steady increase in weight and reps indicates progress and improvement. Moreover, regular strength testing, such as a 1RM test, can help in assessing progress.

5. Body Fat Percentage

Tracking body fat percentage provides a better picture of your body composition. Body fat scales and calipers are inexpensive tools used to track progress. However, it's vital to consider that these tools have a margin of error, and measuring body fat is not always an accurate way to assess progress. Nevertheless, tracking the trend of body fat percentage over time is an essential tool to making informed decisions about adjustments to training and nutrition.

6. Tracking Nutrition

Tracking what you eat with a food diary or journal is also an excellent tool for progress tracking. Recording food intake and monitoring macro and micronutrient intake can point out areas of weakness and help pinpoint potential dietary deficiencies or imbalances.

In conclusion, tracking progress in bodybuilding is not just about the number on a scale or the mirror image. Instead, using a combination of measurements, photos, strength progression, body composition monitoring, and nutrition monitoring will help you get an accurate understanding of your progress. It's crucial to keep measurements consistent and clear to keep tabs on your progress to adjust your plan accordingly to stay motivated and consistent.

POSITIVITY AND MOTIVATION: STAYING FOCUSED ON YOUR BODYBUILDING GOALS

Bodybuilding can be a long and challenging journey, and staying motivated to achieve your goals can be tough. However, maintaining a positive mindset can help keep you focused and motivated throughout your bodybuilding journey. Here are some tips to help you develop positivity and motivation in your bodybuilding journey.

1. Set realistic goals: It's important to set specific, measurable, attainable, relevant, and time-bound (SMART) goals that will help you track progress and celebrate the small victories. Goals like adding 5 pounds to a lift or reducing your body fat percentage by 1% can help keep you motivated.

2. Surround yourself with positive people: The company you keep plays a crucial role in influencing your mindset. Having a supportive and positive group of people around you can help you stay motivated and on track.

3. Visualize your success: It can be beneficial to visualize yourself achieving your bodybuilding goals. Visualizing yourself lifting heavier weights, having a more sculpted physique, or dominating your competition can go a long way in motivating you to keep pushing.

4. Stay consistent: Consistency is key in achieving your bodybuilding goals. Sticking to your workout routine, nutrition plan, and recovery plan can help you stay on track and maintain momentum.

5. Celebrate small victories: Celebrating the small victories, even if they seem small, can help build confidence and motivation. Whether it's lifting heavier weights, achieving a new personal best or losing a half-percent of body fat, recognize and appreciate your accomplishments.

6. Create an uplifting playlist: Music has a powerful impact on our emotions and can influence our mindset. Create a playlist of uplifting and motivational songs that help you stay focused and energized during your workouts.

7. Utilize positive affirmations: Affirmations are positive statements that help us stay focused and motivated. Repeating phrases like "I am capable of achieving my goals," or "I am strong and resilient" can help build self-confidence and positivity.

In summary, staying positive and motivated is essential to achieving your bodybuilding goals. With these tips, you can develop the mindset necessary to stay focused, motivated, and committed to your journey.

HITTING PLATEAUS AND OVERCOMING CHALLENGES IN BODYBUILDING

Anyone who has done bodybuilding for a while knows that progress comes with its share of peaks and plateaus. A plateau in bodybuilding refers to a period of time when you experience little or no progress despite your best efforts. This can be frustrating, and it can lead to a loss of motivation. However, it's important to remember that plateaus are a natural part of the bodybuilding journey. Here are some tips for overcoming them and getting back on track:

1. Change up your routine - Your muscles quickly adapt to the same exercises performed in the same order. Try doing different exercises, changing up the order of your routine, varying your sets and reps, or trying different weights.

2. Increase your weights - Sometimes, you need to increase the resistance to break through a plateau. Try adding 5-10lbs to each exercise or try a weight you've never attempted before.

3. Focus on progressive overload - This technique is essential in continually challenging your muscles from workout to workout, which can help jumpstart progress again. Continue to increase the stress on the body for the muscles to keep getting stronger.

4. Adjust your nutrition - Ensure that you are eating enough protein for your level and directly following your workout. Your body needs the right amount of fuel and micronutrients to build muscle.

5. Reassess your sleep and rest time - Make sure you are getting

7-8 hours of sleep each night and focus on proper rest times during your lifting sessions. Too little sleep and rest time may be contributing to your lack of progress.

6. Seek guidance - If you have been bodybuilding for a while and are still experiencing plateaus, consider hiring a coach or consulting with a nutritionist to help you find areas of improvement.

7. Stay motivated - When you hit a plateau, it's easy to give in to feelings of frustration and self-doubt. Take a step back and remember your reasons for bodybuilding in the first place. Creating a clear image of your goal again and making a plan to achieve it can get you back on track.

Finally, it's important to remember that progress in bodybuilding is not always linear. Some months you will see significant gains, while others are slower. The key is to keep pushing and take a complete approach to your bodybuilding program that outlines your nutrition, workout, and rest habits. By bringing consistency and best practices practices to your program, you can overcome plateaus and ultimately reach your bodybuilding goals.

BODYBUILDING FOR WOMEN: DISPELLING THE MYTHS AND MAXIMIZING RESULTS

Bodybuilding has been perceived as a male-dominated sport for a long time, but it is no longer the case. Women from all over the world are starting to find their place in the gym, fueled by the benefits that weightlifting and bodybuilding routines can offer.

However, there is still a considerable amount of misinformation and myths regarding women and bodybuilding. The aim of this chapter is to dispel those myths and provide tips to help women maximize their results and achieve their goals.

Myth 1: Women should not lift heavy weights

Many women are afraid of lifting heavy weights for fear of becoming too bulky or looking masculine. However, this is not the case. Women have lower testosterone levels compared to men, which makes it nearly impossible for them to get bulky.

On the other hand, lifting heavier weights is beneficial for women's overall health and fitness. It helps build lean muscle mass, increases metabolism, and strengthens bones, reducing the risk of osteoporosis.

Myth 2: Women should focus only on cardio

While cardio exercises such as running, cycling, or swimming are essential for overall cardiovascular health and endurance, they cannot substitute for resistance training, particularly bodybuilding. Cardio helps to burn calories, whereas weightlifting helps to build and shape muscles.

Myth 3: Women need to lift lighter weights and do more reps

Many women incorporate lighter weights into their workout routines to avoid getting too bulky. However, this approach can lead to minimal results. The most effective way to stimulate muscle growth is by lifting heavy weights with fewer reps. Aim for two to three sets of six to ten reps for each exercise.

Myth 4: Women should only train specific body parts

Another common myth is that women should only train specific body parts, such as the glutes or legs. However, muscle development is not localized to specific areas, and training specific muscle groups does not burn more fat in that area.

Instead, engaging in full-body weightlifting and bodybuilding routines will provide the most benefits. Focusing on compound exercises such as squats, deadlifts, and bench presses will target multiple muscle groups simultaneously, leading to increased overall strength, endurance, and muscle mass.

Myth 5: Women should not eat enough protein

Protein is essential for muscle growth and recovery. Consuming adequate protein is crucial for women interested in bodybuilding. Women should aim for 0.8 to 1 gram of protein per pound of body weight. Foods such as eggs, chicken, fish, tofu, and protein shakes can help women meet their daily protein requirements.

In conclusion, women can also benefit significantly from bodybuilding routines, and they shouldn't be afraid of lifting heavy weights. By incorporating weightlifting and bodybuilding into their fitness routine, women can enjoy increased strength, endurance, muscle mass, and overall health.

AGE AND BODYBUILDING: BALANCING SAFETY AND PROGRESSION

As we age, we typically lose muscle mass and strength due to a variety of factors such as a decrease in hormone levels and a more sedentary lifestyle. However, it is never too late to start bodybuilding and reap the many benefits it has to offer.

When it comes to age and bodybuilding, safety is always a top priority. Older adults should consult with a doctor before starting a new exercise program and make sure to properly warm up and cool down to prevent injury.

It is also important to understand that progress in bodybuilding may be slower as we age. Recovery time may be longer and the body may not respond to training as quickly. However, this does not mean that gains cannot be made. With consistency and patience, older adults can still see significant improvements in their physique and overall health.

In terms of training, older adults may benefit from focusing on compound movements that work multiple muscle groups at once, such as squats, deadlifts, and bench presses. These movements can help maintain bone density and promote overall strength and functionality.

Nutrition is also critical for older bodybuilders. Adequate protein intake is essential for muscle growth and repair, and older adults may need to consume slightly more than younger individuals. Additionally, a diet rich in fruits and vegetables can provide important antioxidants and other nutrients to support optimal health.

Bodybuilding can have many benefits for older adults, including improved muscle strength and mobility, increased bone density, and a decreased risk of chronic diseases such as osteoporosis and diabetes. With the right approach and mindset, age is not a barrier to achieving a healthy and strong physique through bodybuilding.

THE SOCIAL AND PSYCHOLOGICAL BENEFITS OF BODYBUILDING

Bodybuilding is not just physical activity but also a mental one. It helps to maintain overall health and well-being. Everyone, regardless
of age, gender, or fitness level, can benefit from bodybuilding. Let us take a closer look at the social and psychological benefits associated with this practice.

1. Boosts Self-confidence: A properly designed bodybuilding program will help you build muscle mass and reduce unwanted fat, resulting in better body shape. This contact with your new look will enhance your confidence and self-esteem. You will feel better about yourself, and that aura of confidence can make an excellent impression on others.

2. Promotes Self-discipline: Getting into a consistent training routine and following a healthy, balanced diet takes a lot of self-discipline. Once you establish a routine, you will be more likely to adhere to it, and those habits will carry over into other areas of your life, such as work or study.

3. Reduces Stress: Exercise is an incredible stress-reliever, and bodybuilding is no exception. Engaging in physical activity releases endorphins, otherwise called the happy hormone. These endorphins can increase feelings of well-being, decrease stress levels, and decrease the risk of anxiety or depression.

4. Enhances Mental Toughness: Bodybuilding is a challenging process, pushing individuals to their limits. It requires a strong mindset to keep going, consistently challenging oneself, and not

giving up during challenging times. This discipline can be applied to other areas of life, creating a well-rounded mentally tough individual.

5. Provides Sense of Accomplishment: Reaching new milestones and achieving fitness goals provides a sense of accomplishment which improves self-esteem and well-being. Seeing consistency in progress and changes is satisfying and increases motivation to keep pushing forward.

6. Helps Build a Supportive Social Circle: Engaging in a bodybuilding routine is an excellent way to meet and connect with like-minded people. It is a great way to socialize and create friendships with people who share similar goals and interests.

In conclusion, bodybuilding has numerous social and psychological benefits. Engaging in this remarkable activity not only improves overall physical fitness but also mental wellness. Building healthy habits in terms of discipline, nutrition, and physical activity can positively affect other areas of life and drastically impact well-being.

COMPETING IN BODYBUILDING: TIPS FOR SUCCESS

Competing in bodybuilding contests can be a grueling and challenging experience, but it can also be immensely rewarding. The discipline and dedication required to prepare for a competition can help you achieve a level of physical and mental fitness that you may have never thought possible. If you're considering entering a bodybuilding contest, here are some tips to help you prepare and succeed:

1. Find a Trusted Coach: Bodybuilding is an art, and like any art, it requires the guidance of a skilled and experienced coach. Finding a coach who understands your goals, your body type, and your training needs is crucial. Your coach will be able to customize a program that works best for you and instruct you on posing, nutrition, and what to expect in the contest.

2. Set Realistic Goals: Competing in a bodybuilding contest requires months of hard work, dedication, and sacrifice. Be sure to set realistic goals for yourself and your training regimen. Competing in a contest is not something you can just decide to do overnight. It takes time, discipline, and a lot of hard work, so be prepared to put in the time and effort necessary.

3. Practice Posing: Posing is an essential component of bodybuilding competitions, and it can make a considerable difference in how you're judged. Practice posing regularly, and make sure you can hold each pose for an extended period. Choose poses that showcase your strengths and downplay your weaknesses.

4. Nail Your Nutrition: Nutrition is a crucial component of

bodybuilding. Your coach will help you create the right diet plan that will work for your specific needs. However, it's essential to understand the basics of sound nutrition on your own. Ensure that you are consuming the right number of calories and macros required to achieve your fitness goals.

5. Train Hard, Train Smart: While consistency is crucial, remember to listen to your body and avoid overdoing it. Overtraining can lead to injuries and setbacks. Vary your workouts, add weights gradually, and take sufficient time to recover after heavy lifts.

6. Be Confident: In a bodybuilding contest, confidence matters. Strut your stuff and focus on showing off what you've worked so hard to achieve. Competing requires not only physical stamina, but also mental endurance.

7. Take Care of Yourself: Competing in a bodybuilding contest can be physically and emotionally draining. You need to ensure that you're getting sufficient sleep, drinking plenty of water, and taking measures to minimize stress.

Competing in a bodybuilding contest can be an incredible experience that shapes you both physically and emotionally. By focusing on the essentials, and building constructive practices around them, you can be better equipped for the challenge, and succeed in building the body you've worked so hard to achieve.

LIFE BEYOND BODYBUILDING: MAINTAINING RESULTS AND HEALTHY HABITS FOR LONG-TERM SUCCESS.

Bodybuilding is much more than just a sport or hobby. It is a lifestyle that requires dedication, hard work, and discipline. However, what happens when you reach your bodybuilding goals? How do you maintain your results and healthy habits for long-term success?

Maintaining Results after Bodybuilding

After months or even years of hard work, dedication, and perseverance, you have finally achieved your dream physique. Congratulations! You should feel proud of yourself for reaching your goal. However, the key to long-term success is to maintain your results.

The first thing to consider is to slowly transition to a maintenance program. You might not need to train as hard or as frequently as you did during the bodybuilding phase, but make sure you find a balance that incorporates strength training, cardio, and recovery.

Incorporating other types of physical activity is also important to maintain your results. Try new activities such as yoga or swimming, and play sports you enjoy. It will help keep you motivated and challenge your body in different ways.

Additionally, make sure you keep your body fueled with proper nutrition. Continue to eat a healthy and well-balanced diet with a good balance of protein, carbs, and fats, and don't forget to stay hydrated. Reducing or completely cutting calories too quickly can lead to muscle loss and a weakened immune system.

Healthy Habits for Long-Term Success

Bodybuilding requires a lot of discipline, and it's essential to maintain healthy habits for long-term success. Here are some tips to keep you on track:

1. Prioritize Sleep: Adequate sleep is essential for muscle recovery, mental focus, and overall health. Aim for 7-8 hours of sleep per night.

2. Reduce Stress: Stress is known to cause muscle breakdown and hinder recovery. Practicing relaxation techniques like meditation or yoga and taking time for self-care are essential to reduce stress levels.

3. Incorporate Cardio: Cardiovascular exercise is essential for heart health and weight management. Aim for at least 150 minutes of moderate-intensity exercise or 75 minutes of high-intensity exercise per week.

4. Stay Positive: A positive mindset is critical to staying motivated and focused on your goals. Surround yourself with supportive and like-minded people who encourage and inspire you.

Conclusion

Bodybuilding is much more than just lifting weights and bulking up muscles. It is a journey that requires discipline, hard work, and dedication. Maintaining your results and healthy habits for long-term success is crucial to live a happy, healthy, and fulfilling life. Remember to find a balance that works for you, stay active, eat well, and take care of your body and mind.